M000107166

Carb Cycling Recipe Book

A Woman's 14 Day Jumpstart Plan

JULIETTE NORTH

<u>Disclaimer Notice:</u>

ISBN: 9781720105725

Contents

Introduction

I want to thank you for purchasing this book, "Carb Cycling Recipe Book: A Woman's 14 Day Jumpstart Plan."

Attention all women: Does the stubborn body fat bother you? Are you tired of all the restrictive diets that claim to be efficient? Do you want to lose fat and weight without giving up on the foods you love? If yes, then this is the perfect book for you.

Carb cycling is the answer to all your prayers. Carb cycling is a simple concept and the protocols of this diet are easy to follow. In this book, you will learn about carb cycling, the benefits of carb cycling, tips to help you along the way, and the ways in which you can develop a carb cycling plan for yourself. You will also find recipes to cook delicious and nutritious food according to the carb requirement.

Not only will you lose weight, but you can effectively keep it at bay as well. So, if you are ready, then let us start without further ado!

CHAPTER 1: ABOUT CARB CYCLING

If you want to lose weight, build muscle, lose fat, and get into shape then the best tool at your disposal is carb cycling. Carb cycling is quite simple, provided you know what you need to do. In this section, you will learn what carb cycling is all about.

Before you learn about carb cycling, you need to know what carbs are. So, what are carbs or carbohydrates? Carbohydrates refer to the sugars that the human body uses to generate energy. Carbs consist of different components like sugars, starches, and fiber or cellulose. The human body uses two sources of energy and these are glucose and fatty acids that are present in our diets. Carbs are responsible for the surge of energy or quick energy and are simplified into muscle or liver glycogen that's stored in the body. When you indulge in any form of high-intensity exercise like resistance training, sprinting, bodyweight training or any other form of exercise that requires a lot of energy in short bursts, the body dips into its stores of carbs for fuel.

Carb cycling is a simple dieting protocol wherein you need to consume high levels of carbs on certain days and follow it up with low or no-carb days. The simplest explanation is that on some days you will eat lots of carbs and on other days you will eat less or no carbs.

Carb cycling is a strategic method to set up your diet. If you want to use this method to lose weight, lose fat, gain muscle or improve your overall performance, then it is important that you do it properly. The way you design your diet is pretty much up to you, your goals, and your dietary choices. Here are a couple of things that you must know before we delve further into this topic.

There are different ways in which you can follow this diet. There is no single right or wrong manner to go about carb cycling. Some prefer to consume a high-carb diet on most of the days whereas others might opt for a low-carb diet. Regardless of your goals (fat loss, maintenance of weight, weight loss, muscle gain or anything else), you can use the method of carb cycling.

The main purpose of carb cycling is to help you make the most of your body composition and training. If you carefully monitor your carb intake daily, it is easier to manage your calorie deficit or surplus, depending on your goal. Carb cycling tries to manipulate the stores of glycogen in the body in a strategic method by topping up the body's stores of carbs to replace all that are used during exercise. For instance, athletes tend to consume high-carb meals the night before a marathon or a race. They consume plenty of carbs to make sure that the stores of glycogen in their body are full. In this manner, they will have plenty of glycogen to generate energy from on the following day.

At present, there isn't a lot of research that explains the science behind carb cycling. Most of the studies about diets focus on the effect of food on the body in terms of its contribution towards health instead of performance and body composition. Carb cycling is a simple concept.

Here are all the things that the high-carb days

are meant for:

- Refill the stores of muscle glycogen in the body

- To improve overall performance

- Increase the production of hormones like leptin that trigger hunger cues

- Any spare protein to reduce the breakdown of muscles from intensive training and carb restriction

Here are all the things that the low-carb days are meant for:

- To induce calorie deficit in order to help the body burn fat

- To control calorie intake to facilitate weight loss

- Manage any spikes in insulin levels

Carb cycling is an ideal meal plan if you want any or all of the following:

- Gain muscle without a proportional increase in fat

- Gain and maintain a lean body frame

- To lose fat without any loss of muscle

- Improve insulin sensitivity in your body

Apart from this, carb cycling is an ideal diet for all those who want to include a variety of macros in their diet and want to enjoy carb-rich and fatty meals. If you want all this or any of these things, then carb cycling is the best diet for you.

Carb cycling will help you manage hunger pangs and will help you adhere to the diet since you will feel full from the strategically spaced high-carb days followed by low-carb days. It will improve your body's ability to store glycogen and help build muscle. It also helps you retain lean muscle by ensuring that the glycogen stores in the body are regularly replenished. Apart from this, it also regulates the secretion of leptin. Leptin is a hunger hormone, the higher the level of leptin, the fuller you will feel. You will learn more about the different benefits of this diet in the coming chapters.

The only thing that you must be wary of when you try this diet is to control your impulse to binge on unhealthy junk food on the high-carb days. If you maintain or cultivate a healthy relationship with food, then you don't have to worry about it. Don't try to compensate for the low-carb or no-carb days on the days that you can eat carbs. If you alternate between days of restriction and binging on junk, you will not be doing yourself any favors. Show some restraint and eat healthily. To eat healthy, delicious and nutritious food on all days, go through the recipes curated in this book. Anyone can follow this diet. However, if you suffer from any eating disorders or are recovering from any eating disorders, then please refrain from following this diet.

CHAPTER 2: METHOD OF CARB CYCLING

There are various ways in which you can implement carb cycling. In general, a regular carb cycling diet includes high-carb, low-carb and no carb days.

High-Carb Days

On a typical high-carb day, more than 50% or even the total carb intake will be in the form of starch and fruits. The kind of carbs you consume will depend on your requirements, goals, and the level of activity. The number of carbs you consume can be anywhere between

2-4 times your body weight in grams of carbs. For instance, if you weigh about 120 pounds, then your carb consumption on a high-carb day can be anywhere between:

120 x 2 = 240 grams to 120 x 4 = 480 grams of carbs. If you feel that 480 grams of carbs are too much, well, that's because it is. You must opt for the highest carb consumption, only if you engage in high-intensity training that requires a lot of energy. Eat carbs according to your schedule. If cardio is the only exercise you plan on doing, then you certainly don't need 480 grams of carbs. 240 grams of carbs is sufficient enough.

Medium-Carb Days

On a typical low-carb day, your carb intake will be roughly 25-50% of your total consumption of macros. For the sake of numbers, you can consume 0.5 grams to 1.5 grams of carbs per pound of your weight. So, your carb consumption on a low-carb day can be anywhere in between:

120 x 0.5 = 60 grams to 120 x 1.5 = 180 grams

of carbs. The amount of carbs is based on the total caloric requirement and the number can vary. On a low-carb day, most of your carbs will be in the form of green vegetables and some fruit. These sources of carbs are more filling than other starchy foods.

Low Carb Day

On a no carb day, your total carb intake will probably be less than 10% of your total calorie intake. You can consume anywhere between 0 to 50 grams of carbs. Practically, it might not be possible to have 0 grams of carb, unless you plan to eat nothing other than meat and fatty foods. Most people on a no carb day tend to include green and fibrous vegetables for some carbs. Not to sound like a broken record, but there is no right or wrong way to go about carb cycling. In fact, the key factor to consider is your personal preferences, your needs, and requirements. Some people can vary their intake daily and then there are those that cannot do so. For most people, the protein intake will usually be static. Your protein intake needs to be between 0.8 to 1 gram per pound of your body weight. For instance, a 120-pound woman will need to consume anywhere between 96 to 120 grams of protein daily. If you want to maintain your muscle mass, then it is ideal to consume 1 gram of protein per pound of body weight. The total fat you consume will be between 15 to 35% of your total calorie intake per day.

Methods

There are different approaches that you can adopt for carb cycling. The most popular ones are as follows:

The Zigzag Method

Day 1- Low carb with light to moderate exercise

Day 2- No carbs and rest

Day 3- High carb with intensive training

Day 4- No carbs and rest

Day 5- Low carb with light to moderate

exercise

Day 6- High carb with intensive training

Day 7- Repeat the entire process again

Every Other Day Method

Day 1- Low carb or no carb and rest day

Day 2- High carbs and intensive exercise or training

Day 3- Low carb or no carb and rest day

Day 4- High carbs and intensive exercise or training

Day 5- Low carb or no carb and rest day

Day 6- High carbs and intensive exercise or training

Day 7- Low carb or no carb and rest day

Then start with a high carb day and repeat the same process.

Weekly Carb Re-Feed Method

Day 1- Low carb intake and mild training or exercise

Day 2- No carbs and rest

Day 3- Low carb intake and mild training or exercise

Day 4- No carbs and rest

Day 5- Low carb intake and mild training or exercise

Day 6- No carbs and rest

Day 7- High carbohydrate intake. You can either rest or train on this day according to your body's ability to recover and replenish the glycogen stores.

Fat Loss and Muscle Gain

One question that a lot of people seem to have is whether carb cycling helps with fat loss. If you are wondering the same, then the answer is yes. Carb cycling is a good approach to lose fat. However, you need to keep a simple thing in mind. You cannot lose fat unless your body is on a calorie deficit. You need to make sure that your body burns more calories than the number of calories you consume. If there is no calorie deficit, then you cannot lose fat. So, how does carb cycling help with fat loss? The strategic pattern of eating carbs allows you to fill up on carbs on certain days so that you feel full even on a calorie deficit. It will help you maintain your performance while exercising and training. A restriction on carb consumption encourages your body to burn stored fat to provide energy.

The next question is does carb cycling helps with muscle gain or not? Yes, carb cycling helps with muscle gain as well. There are a couple of factors that trigger muscle gain. To gain muscle, you need to maintain a calorie surplus, give your body the necessary time to rest and recover from intensive training and engage in a little resistance training. You need to understand one thing about your body. You can either gain muscle or lose fat. However, you cannot do both of these things simultaneously. Think about it, you cannot maintain calorie surplus as well as calorie deficit at the same time, can you? So, your diet will primarily depend on your health and fitness goals. If you want to gain muscle, then strategically feed your body with carbs to increase the muscle mass. Another thing that you must be aware of is that a calorie surplus also leads to fat gain. Regardless of how you go about it, if you want to develop muscle mass, some fat comes along with it. There is no special macronutrient ratio to avoid this situation. Therefore, it is prudent that you manage your total calorie surplus in such a manner that you don't gain more weight than necessary.

CHAPTER 3 – WHAT TO EAT?

In this section, you will learn about the different foods that you can and cannot eat if you want to follow carb cycling.

High-Carb Days

On a high carb day, your main focus will be on carb-rich foods like fruits, vegetables, tubers and different grains. The portion of fatty foods you consume will be low and you need to opt for lean sources of protein.

The ideal sources of carbs include rice, bread, pasta, potatoes, any of the vegetables you like, and all fruits. Ideal sources of fat include trace fats from different sources like eggs, meat, fish and so on. For protein, you can include lean cuts of beef and pork, chicken, and fish. If you want to include dairy products then opt for lean dairy products like low-fat milk, yogurt, and cheese. You can include some whey protein or pea protein shakes as well.

Medium-Carb Days

On medium-carb days your main focus needs to be on carbohydrate sources that are low in carbs and will satiate your hunger like tubers, vegetables, and certain fruits. To compensate for the reduction in the carbs, you can include naturally fatty foods on moderate carb days.

The ideal sources of carbs include potatoes, green and fibrous vegetables, and some fruits (like berries, melons and don't include fruit juices). You can include fatty cuts of meats, eggs, and full-fat dairy products. You can include fatty and non-fatty dairy sources, whey protein, pea protein and even lean cuts of meat.

Low-Carb Days

Your carb intake on a low-carb day must not exceed 50 grams. Your main focus on a low-carb day will be green vegetables. In fact, green and fibrous vegetables are the only sources of carbs that you can include in your diet. You can include fatty cuts of meat (beef, pork, and lamb) and full-fat dairy products (milk, cheese, and yogurt).

Meal Timing

Meal timing in carb cycling is subject to your discretion. There are two things that your meal timings depend on and these are your preferred meal timings and your ability to consume the necessary calories for the day. For instance, if you need to consume 3000 calories on a training day, then it probably isn't easy to consume all the calories in one huge meal. You cannot fast all day long and indulge in one heavy meal during intensive training. It is not ideal because your muscles need some time to synthesize all the carbs and protein you consume. In such a case, you can consume three to four meals during the day. You can easily distribute your calorie intake throughout the day. On a low-carb day, you can perhaps have two meals and one snack between each meal. It is up to you and the plan you design for yourself. If you want to build muscle, then you need to eat at regular intervals instead of one large meal at the end of the day.

Glycogen is of two types and it includes muscle glycogen and liver glycogen. All starchy carbs like grains, potatoes, bread, pasta, and the like are stored within the body in the form of muscle glycogen; whereas fructose from fruits, juices, and simple sugars help refill the levels of liver glycogen in the body. On a high-carb day, your aim is to replenish the level of muscle glycogen and on low-carb days, you need to replenish your liver glycogen stores.

CHAPTER 4 – BENEFITS OF CARB CYCLING

In this section, you will learn about the different benefits of a carb cycling diet.

Build and Preserve Lean Muscle

Different forms of resistance and strength training breakdown the existing muscle tissue and build it back stronger. A lot of energy is necessary to rebuild and repair existing tissue in the body. The primary fuel necessary for this process comes from the carbs that you consume. After working out, carbs restore the energy levels in the body and provide the muscles with the necessary glycogen to rebuild the muscles. If you don't consume sufficient calories and carbs after resistance training, then it is quite likely that you will starve your muscles of the fuel that they need to rebuild themselves. This is the primary reason why a lot of people opt for heavy and intensive training on high carb days.

If you simply restrict your calorie intake and work out more than what your metabolism can sustain, it will have the opposite of the effect you desire. If you train intensively and don't provide your body with the necessary fuel it needs to sustain itself, you will feel weak and tired. It is a good idea to alternate between days of high and low carb intake, especially when you time your workouts according to your intake of carbohydrates. When you follow the protocols of carb cycling, you will be able to maintain your muscle mass and lose fat too. Your body gets sufficient time to restore and replenish its stores of energy and it doesn't have to burn any of the muscle mass for the sake of energy.

Maintenance of Weight Loss

Not only does carb cycling help with weight loss, it also helps you maintain the weight loss. It is effective because this diet allows you to eat the foods that you love, and you don't have to give up on anything, unlike most fad diets. Instead, it is all about eating strategically to achieve your weight loss and health goals.

Reduce Fluctuations in Blood Sugar Levels

All the carbohydrates that you consume are broken down into simple sugars during digestion. When this happens, the simple sugars are free to enter the bloodstream and this leads to an increase in the level of your blood sugar. A high level of blood sugar is toxic, and the body starts to release a hormone called insulin. Insulin helps in breaking down these simple sugars into glucose and transports these to different cells. The cells then burn this glucose for generating energy. When an individual is healthy, a spike in the blood sugar is counteracted by the production of insulin and there's no damage.

CHAPTER 5 – SMART CARB CYCLING

Before you learn to structure a carb cycling plan, you need to determine the ideal macronutrient breakdown for your body.

Step 1: Macronutrient Breakdown

Protein Intake

If you want to maintain your muscle mass while you restrict the intake of calories, then you need to feed your body sufficient protein. Your body needs about 0.8 to 1.2 grams of protein per pound of fat-free mass in your body. If you are lean and have been restricting your calorie intake for longer, then your protein intake needs to be higher up the scale. The opposite is true if you have more body fat. People usually follow a simple "body weight X 1" calculation to find their protein intake. However, a better idea is to multiply one gram of protein with your fat-free body mass. For instance, if your weight is 120 lbs and you have 15% body fat, then your body fat accounts for (120 x 0.15) 18 lbs of body fat. In that case, your lean body mass is (120-18) 102 lbs. To determine your daily protein intake, you need to multiply 1.2 grams of protein with your lean body mass. Therefore, your protein intake needs to be between 100 to 122 grams of protein per day.

Fat Intake

About 20 to 25% of your total calorie intake needs to be in the form of dietary fats. It means that you need to consume anywhere between 0.3 to 0.4 grams of fat per pound of your bodyweight. If you weigh 120 pounds, then your daily fat intake will be between 36 to 48 grams (bodyweight X 0.4 grams) of fat.

Carb Intake

If you are a physically active person, then you must never avoid carbohydrates. Carbohydrates are the main source of fuel for the body. When you overfeed, they are stored in the form of fat within the body cells. You need to consume carbs in such a manner that it will allow you to stay in a deficit. A good place to start will be to multiply 1 to 1.5 grams of carbs by your bodyweight to find your daily intake of carbs.

So, your daily carb intake will be 120 to 180 grams of carbs.

Step 2: Weekly Intake of Carbs and Fats

Using the previous example of a 120-pound woman, you need to start your diet with about 120 grams of protein, 50 grams of fat, and about 180 grams of carbs. One gram of fat contains 9 calories. One gram of protein and carb contains 4 calories each. Therefore, your daily calorie intake will be as follows:

120 x 4 = 480 calories from protein

50 x 9 = 450 calories from fat

180 x 4 = 720 calories from carbohydrates

Your daily calorie intake is around 1650 kcal per day and about 11,500 kcal per week. As long as you can ensure that you consume 1650 kcal per week or less than that, your body will be in a deficit and you will lose fat. You will lose fat regardless of the carb distribution in the week.

It means that you will consume about 350 grams of fat and 1260 grams of carbs per week. The idea is to manipulate your diet while you stay within the above numbers to improve your performance and lose weight at the same time. The better your performance is the less likely it is that you will lose muscle mass.

Step 3: High, Moderate and Low Carb Days

The next step is to determine your high-carb, moderate carb, and low carb days in a week. It is quite easy to determine these days. All the days that you engage in high-intensity training need to be high carb days, for medium intensity training you need moderate carbs and on the days you rest, your body can do with low or no carbs. So, you can have two days of intensive training, two medium sessions, and three days to recover from all the exercise. Now that you are aware of your training program, you need to distribute your carb intake accordingly.

On the days of intensive training, you will cover about 50% of your weekly carb intake, 35% for your moderate sessions and the rest 15% on your rest days. For instance, if your weekly carb intake needs to be 1260 grams, then your carb intake will be as follows.

On high carb days, you will consume 50% of your total weekly carbs. It means that for two high-carb days your total carb intake will be 630 carbs (for two days). On the days of moderate training or medium-carb days, your carb intake will be 440 carbs (two days). The rest, 189 grams of carbs you can consume on your rest days (three days in a week).

Your carb intake on a high-carb day is 315

grams. The carb intake on a moderate carb day is 220 grams and that on the rest day or low-carb day is 63 grams.

Step 4: High, Moderate and Low-Fat Days

Your total fat consumption in a week needs to be 350 grams.

You need to follow the same strategy to distribute your weekly fat intake as well.

On the days of high-intensity training, your fat intake needs to be low. On days of moderate training, your fat intake needs to be moderate. On the other days, your fat intake needs to be high. The two days of the week during which your carb intake is high, you need to consume 15% (52.5 grams) of your weekly fat. On the moderate training days in the week, you need to consume 25% (88 grams) of your weekly fats and the rest of the fat (210 grams) on the no or low-carb days.

Your fat intake on a high-fat day is 70 grams of fat. Your fat intake on a moderate fat day is 44 grams and that on a low-fat day is 26 grams.

Here is a sample of the weekly breakdown of macronutrients that you need:

Day	Carbohydrate	Protein	Fat
Monday (High intensity)	315 grams High Carb	100-120 grams	26 grams Low fat
Tuesday (Moderate intensity)	220 grams Moderate Carb	100-120 grams	44 grams Moderate fat
Wednesday (Rest)	50-63 grams Low-Carb	100-120 grams	70 grams High fat
Thursday (High intensity)	315 grams High Carb	100-120 grams	26 grams Low fat
Friday (Moderate intensity)	220 grams Moderate Carb	100-120 grams	44 grams Moderate fat

Saturday (Rest)	5 0 - 6 3 grams Low-Carb	1 0 0-1 2 0 grams	70 grams High fat
Sunday (Rest)	5 0 - 6 3 grams Low-Carb	1 0 0-1 2 0 grams	70 grams High fat

Here are the different forms of exercise that you can opt for when you follow the protocols of carb cycling. Each type of exercise has a different nutritional need. There are four different types of exercises - aerobic, anaerobic, flexibility, and stability.

- Aerobic exercise: Anything that lasts over three minutes is an aerobic exercise, which is also known as cardio. Steady state cardio with low intensity helps burn fat.

- Anaerobic exercise: High-intensity interval training or weight training by shorter bursts of energy is anaerobic exercise. Fat alone cannot provide enough energy because carbs are the primary fuel for these exercises. Include this form of exercise on a high-carb day.

- Flexible exercise: Injuries caused by shortening of the muscles can be prevented by increasing flexibility of the body so these exercises help in improving muscle range of the body, supporting joints and stretching your muscle. The best examples are after work-out stretches and yoga.

- Stability exercise: control of movement, improving alignment and stretching of muscles can be achieved by these exercises, which generally include balance exercises and core training.

CHAPTER 6 – ANY HEALTH CONCERNS

If you want to try carb cycling, then there are certain things that you need to keep in mind.

Never Ignore your Thyroid

The thyroid is an essential hormone for fat loss. However, on a low carb diet, the production of thyroid will slow down in the body. When the production of thyroid slows down, it can cause problems with a woman's metabolic system. Women are more sensitive to the behavior of the thyroid than men. An imbalance in the thyroid hormone can lead to hypothyroidism.

So, how can you avoid it? It is quite simple. You need to make sure that your body gets at least 50 grams of carbs on any given day. It is quite easy to include 50 grams of carbs in your daily meal. Never scrimp on carbs, if you don't want to harm your thyroid secretion in the body. Did you know that something as simple as one large sweet potato contains 50 grams of carbs?

Menstrual Cycle

Two hormones that influence carbohydrate metabolism in women are estrogen and progesterone. Estrogen can increase insulin sensitivity and progesterone tends to decrease insulin sensitivity in the body. During the first two weeks of the cycle or the follicular phase, the body can process carbs more efficiently than during the last two weeks of the cycle. The last two weeks of the cycle are the ones after ovulation and during this period, when the body starts to process carbs, most of it is stored in the form of fat in the body. Therefore, be mindful of your menstrual cycle while you decide the low and the high carb days. If you place most of your high carb days during the last two weeks of your monthly cycle, your body will not burn carbs efficiently and it will lead to fat gain in the body.

Starvation Mode

When you opt for carb cycling, you need to ensure that your diet lets you consume a sufficient amount of calories. Most women tend to think that a low-calorie diet is more effective than other forms of diet. If you don't consume sufficient calories and skimp on carbs while you exercise, then it will harm your body's ability to regulate the reproductive hormones in your body. If you skimp on calories as well as carbs, then your body can misinterpret this as external stress. While under stress, the body shuts down the reproductive system. It doesn't matter if this so-called "stress" is voluntary. Your body cannot differentiate between a self-imposed calorie deficit and one caused due to starvation. It will affect your reproductive health if you aren't mindful of all that you eat.

A woman's body is relatively more sensitive to

the signals of starvation than that of a man. So, whenever your body notices a decrease in your food intake, it tends to misinterpret the same as starvation and in turn, increases the production of leptin and ghrelin. Leptin and ghrelin are the two hormones that trigger hunger. When there is an increase in the secretion of these chemical compounds, you will experience extreme hunger. Technically, your body doesn't need any extra food, but it is merely your hormones that tell you otherwise. Whenever a woman's body feels that it is headed towards a famine (intentional or not), it increases the secretion of the hunger hormones. The hunger hormones, as is obvious from the name, signal your body to increase the intake of food. Also, if there isn't enough food to survive, then your body will start to shut its reproductive system. A woman's body will not want to procreate when it feels like there isn't sufficient sustenance to nourish itself. In fact, it is the body's natural defense against a potential pregnancy during famines. Your body will protect itself from pregnancy, regardless of whether you want to conceive or not. Your body cannot differentiate between a self-imposed fast and a famine. Therefore, the body cannot differentiate between starvation and calorie reduction. That is why the default protective mechanism kicks in.

CHAPTER 7 – HELPFUL TIPS

Human bodies are quite efficient. You can adapt your body to different training programs within no time. If there is no change in physical stimuli, then your body tends to stay the same. However, if you eat the same foods all the time, it will hit a plateau in your progress. The best manner in which you can encourage your body to change is to periodically alter your diet. If you want your body to burn fats to provide energy or create a meal plan that better suits your energy needs, then carb cycling is the simple answer. Carb cycling is simple and all that you need to do is alter your carb intake daily. In this section, you will learn about a couple of tips that will help you along the way.

Don't Skip Meals

Do you tend to skip meals? Regardless of how busy you might be, you always have the time for a quick meal. Don't skip any meals. Your body needs glucose to function and glucose is obtained by breaking down the carbs that you consume. So, when you skip a meal, you are denying your body the fuel that it needs to function, and this leads to imbalances in your blood sugar levels. When your blood sugar is low, you will feel dizzy and lightheaded. It also affects your mood. When your brain doesn't get sufficient glucose, it cannot function optimally. It can lead to mood swings and you will be irritable. You can easily remedy this; you just need to make it a point to eat. Skipping meals increases your risk of diabetes. It happens because of the delay in your body's response to processing insulin when you don't have timely meals. All this is bound to harm your metabolism. When you skip meals, your body automatically shifts into starvation mode and starts slowing down its metabolism. If you are trying to lose weight by skipping meals, you are merely sabotaging your weight loss program. It leads to acid reflux and can result in ulcers and severe abdominal pain.

Don't Overeat

You need to have well-balanced meals. You must not skip your meals, but this doesn't mean that you need to overeat either. Eat only when you are hungry and stop yourself from eating unnecessarily. Here are a couple of simple things that you can do to avoid overeating.

Learn to eat slowly. It certainly isn't a new concept but not many follow it. We are all in a hurry these days. Take a moment and slow down. Take a sip of water between bites and chew your food thoroughly before swallowing it. Don't just gulp down your food; learn to chew it slowly. Start paying attention to what you are eating. Savor the food you are eating and don't just stuff yourself with food. Think about the different textures and flavors. Savor every bite you eat and make it a pleasurable experience. Make your first bites count and satisfy your taste buds. Make use of a smaller plate, this will enable you to control the portions you eat visually thinking you have already eaten enough as opposed to using a larger plate. Stay away from foods that are rich in calories but do nothing to satisfy your appetite. Choose foods that will fill you up; foods that are satisfying. Foods rich in protein and fiber will fill your tummy. Instead of having a bar of chocolate or a pint of ice cream, have a portion of meat with grilled vegetables. This will satiate your hunger. Food that is rich in calories makes you feel full for a while but you will be hungry within an hour. This results in overeating. By being mindful of what you are eating, you can stop yourself from overeating. While eating, make it a point to stay away from all electronic gadgets. This means no television or mobile gadgets. The next time you are bored, don't reach out for the box of cookies or the bag of chips. Think before indulging in mindless eating, the results will be worth it!

Drink Plenty of Water

Water is good for your body and drinking plenty of water will make your skin clearer and will flush out all of the toxins from your body.

Make it a habit to have at least 8 glasses of water daily. If you want to, you can add some flavorings or electrolytes to your water to spruce it up. Slices of lemon, different berries, a handful of mint leaves, or slices of cucumber can be added to water for making detox water. By following these five simple tips, you can trick yourself into drinking water.

Drinking water needs to be convenient. Carry a water bottle or a sipper with yourself wherever you go. If a water bottle is handy, it is more likely that you will drink water without a reminder. Instead of sugary sodas and sweetened beverages, you can have unsweetened water-based drinks. Instead of a Frappuccino, have a cup of Americano. Make it a point to drink a glass of water before and after your meals. Set a goal and measure the amount of water you are drinking daily. If you keep a track of your water intake, you will be motivated to drink more. Don't forget to drink water even when you go out drinking with your friends. Don't let your body get dehydrated.

Whole Grains are Good for You

At least half of the grains you consume must be whole-grains. Examples of whole grains are barley, brown rice, oatmeal, popcorn, bulgur, buckwheat, and millet. Replace the regular grains you consume with whole grains and wholegrain products. Instead of regular pasta, buy wholegrain pasta. It tastes the same and is much better for your health. Check the labels before you buy something to make sure that you are buying wholegrain produce. These grains help in improving your heart's health, can reduce the risk of certain cancers, quite helpful in managing diabetes, and helps in managing your weight as well.

Be Mindful of What You Eat

Always make sure that you increase the intake of leafy vegetables on low-carb days. Leafy greens are rich in fiber and it will make you feel fuller for a longer period of time. Even if your calorie intake is low, you will not feel hungry if you fill yourself up with a generous serving of leafy greens. On the low-carb days, your main source of energy will be from whole-foods. Whole foods include foods that are naturally full of healthy fats like avocados, eggs, coconut oil, fish caught in the wild, nuts and grass-fed butter.

You need to measure your intake of fats and carbs. If you want to stick to carb cycling, then it is important that you stay within the ideal levels of proper carb and fat intake. It will not do your body any good if you overestimate your carb intake and underestimate the intake of protein.

If you want to reduce your carb intake on moderate-carb and low-carb days, then you need to increase your intake of fats. You must never eliminate one macronutrient without substituting it with another source. Your body needs either fats or carbs to generate energy. If you deplete your body of both the sources of energy, it will shift to starvation mode. Be mindful of the macros you feed your body on the days you exercise.

Keep these simple tips in mind when you follow carb cycling. It will certainly make your diet much more effective.

CHAPTER 8 – SAMPLE PLAN

Here is a sample of a week of carb cycling. According to your goal, you can follow any of the carb cycling patterns discussed in this chapter.

Day and Goal (Exercise)	Fat Loss	Gain Mass	Weight maintenance
	(To lose fat your carb intake needs to be low on the days you train and on the other days it needs to be moderate)	(Your carb intake needs to be high on all those days that you train the major muscle groups)	(On the days that you don't train, your carb intake needs to be low to prevent fat gain)

Monday (Chest and triceps)	Low carb day (0.5 grams per pound)	Medium carb day	Medium carb day
		Medium carb day (1.5 grams per pound)	Medium carb day (1.5 grams per pound)
Tuesday (Back and biceps)	Low carb day (0.5 grams per pound)	High carb day (2.5 grams per pound)	Medium carb day
			Medium carb day (1.5 grams per pound)
Wednesday (Rest)	Medium carb day (1.5 grams per pound)	Low carb day (0.5 grams per pound)	Low carb day (0.5 grams per pound)
Thursday (Legs)	Low carb day (0.5 grams per pound)	High carb day (2.5 grams per pound)	Medium carb day
			Medium carb day (1.5 grams per pound)

Friday (Delts and arms)	Low carb day (0.5 grams per pound)	Medium carb day Medium carb day (1.5 grams per pound)	Medium carb day Medium carb day (1.5 grams per pound)
Saturday (Rest)	Low carb day (0.5 grams per pound)	Low carb day (0.5 grams per pound)	Low carb day (0.5 grams per pound)
Sunday (Rest)	Medium carb day Medium carb day (1.5 grams per pound)	Low carb day (0.5 grams per pound)	Low carb day (0.5 grams per pound)

Carb Cycling Sample Menu

Here is a sample of a carb cycling menu:

High-Carb Day

Breakfast

You can include 3 boiled eggs or any other style of whole eggs, 3 slices of multigrain bread, a portion of mushrooms, a side of roasted tomatoes and a bowl of mixed fruit. It will all come up to about 60 grams of carbs.

Lunch

For lunch, you can have 6oz of any lean meat or fish of your choice, along with 6 oz of sweet potatoes or any similar starch and a side of mixed vegetables. The total carb count in this meal is around 45 grams.

Pre-workout snack

A scoop of whey protein, one serving of oatmeal with almond milk or regular milk and a cup of berries of your choice. The total carb count in this meal comes up to 50 grams.

Dinner

One serving of unpolished rice, 6 oz of lean

meat, homemade tomato sauce, a portion of kidney beans and a bowl of mixed vegetables. This meal adds up to 70 grams of carbs.

Medium-Carb Day

Breakfast

One cup of grass-fed yogurt that is high in protein with a cup of mixed berries and a spoonful of mixed seeds. It adds up to 25 grams of carbs.

Lunch

You can have 6 ounces of chicken salad with a 4oz side of diced potatoes. It adds up to 25 grams of carbs.

Pre-workout snack

Have one banana with a weigh protein shake. It adds up to 30 grams of carbs.

Dinner

You can have a serving of sweet potato fries, with 6oz of lean beef, some homemade tomato sauce, one portion of kidney beans and a serving of mixed vegetables. It sums up to approximately 40 grams of carbohydrates.

Low-Carb Day

Breakfast

Have three eggs with three slices of bacon and a portion of mixed vegetables. Your breakfast needs to have about 10 grams of carbs.

Lunch

It can include 6oz of salmon salad (without skin) along with an olive oil dressing. The total carbs are about 10 grams.

Snack

Have 1 oz of mixed nuts with one serving of turkey slice or turkey jerky. The total carbs in your snack are about 10 grams.

Dinner

For dinner, you can have a 6 oz lean steak with half an avocado and a portion of mixed vegetables. The total carbs you consume for dinner at this meal is about 16 grams. On a low-carb day, ensure that your total carb intake does not exceed 50 grams.

Scrambled Eggs with Vegetables (Low Carb)

Serves: 2

Nutritional values per serving:

Calories – 338, Fat – 27 g, Carbohydrate – 8 g, Protein – 17 g

Image Courtesy: Pixabay

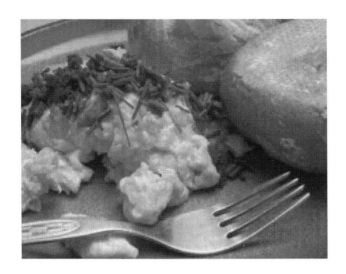

Ingredients:

- 4 teaspoons olive oil

- 1 large clove garlic, minced

- 4 large eggs

- ¼ teaspoon salt

- 2 tablespoons cheddar or gouda cheese, shredded

- 1 cup broccoli, chopped

- 1 cup zucchini, chopped

- 1 teaspoon fresh rosemary, minced

- 2 tablespoons heavy cream

- ½ teaspoon pepper powder

Method:

1. Place a skillet over medium heat. Add oil. When the oil is heated, add broccoli and zucchini and sauté until tender.

2. Add garlic and rosemary and sauté for a few seconds until fragrant.

3. Add eggs, cream, salt, and pepper into a bowl and whisk well. Pour into the skillet. Mix well. Stir frequently until the eggs are nearly cooked.

4. Stir in the cheese and remove the skillet from heat. Mix well.

5. Divide into 2 plates and serve.

Oatmeal with Flax and Chia (High Carb)

Serves: 2

Nutritional values per serving:

Calories – 350, Fat – 14 g, Carbohydrate – 34 g, Protein – 20 g

Image Courtesy: Pixabay

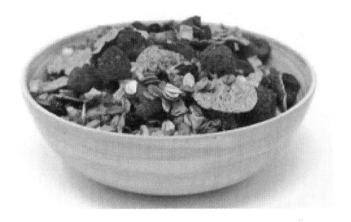

Ingredients:

- 1 1/3 cups raspberries, divided
- 4 tablespoons chia seeds
- 6 tablespoons flax seed meal
- 1 cup nonfat plain Greek yogurt

- 1 teaspoon vanilla extract

- ½ teaspoon liquid stevia

- 1 cup almond milk, unsweetened

- 1 teaspoon cinnamon powder

Method:

1. Add half the raspberries into a bowl. Mash with a fork. Add chia seeds, flax seed meal, yogurt, vanilla, stevia, almond milk, and cinnamon. Mix well.

2. Add remaining half of the raspberries and fold gently.

3. Cover and chill for 4-8 hours.

4. Divide into 2 bowls and serve.

Smoked Salmon Breakfast Wraps (Low Carb)

Serves: 2

Nutritional values per serving: 1 wrap

Calories – 124, Fat – 6 g, Carbohydrate – 14 g, Protein – 12 g

Image Courtesy: Pixabay

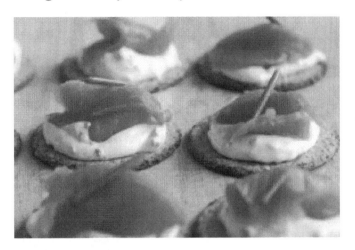

Ingredients:

- 3 tablespoons light cream cheese spread

- 2 teaspoons lemon zest, finely shredded

- 2 whole wheat flour tortillas (6-7 inches)

- ½ small zucchini, trimmed, peeled into ribbons

- ½ tablespoon fresh snipped chives

- 2 teaspoons lemon juice

- 1.5 ounces smoked salmon, thinly sliced, cut into strips

- Lemon wedges to serve (optional)

Method:

1. Add cream cheese, lemon juice, lemon zest and chives into a bowl and stir.

2. Place tortillas on a serving platter. Spread the cream cheese mixture over the tortillas. Do not spread on the edges of the tortillas.

3. Place half the salmon on one-half of the tortillas. Top the salmon with half the zucchini ribbons. Roll from the filled side.

4. Place a wrap in each plate along with a lemon wedge and serve.

Rainbow Frittata (Low Carb)

Serves: 2

Nutritional values per serving: 2 wedges

Calories – 219, Fat – 15 g, Carbohydrate – 8 g, Protein – 14 g

Image Courtesy: Pixabay

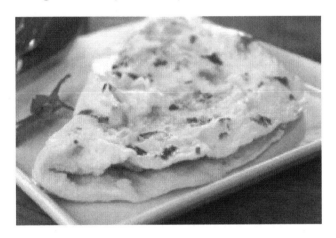

Ingredients:

- 1/8 cup sweet potatoes, chopped

- 1/8 cup broccoli, chopped

- ½ teaspoon fresh basil, chopped

- Freshly cracked pepper to taste

- 2 ¾ cups grape or cherry tomatoes, halved

- Nonstick cooking spray

- 1/8 cup yellow bell pepper, chopped

- 4 omega-3 enriched eggs

- ¼ teaspoon snipped fresh thyme

- ½ avocado, peeled, sliced

- Salt to taste

- Sriracha sauce to taste

Method:

1. Place an ovenproof skillet over medium heat. Spray with cooking spray.

2. When the pan is heated, stir in the bell pepper, sweet potato, and broccoli and sauté until tender. Stir occasionally.

3. Add eggs into a bowl. Whisk well. Add thyme, basil, pepper, and salt and whisk well.

4. Pour into the pan. Do not stir. In a

while, the eggs will begin to set. Gently lift the edges with a spatula to allow the raw egg to reach below.

5. Turn off the heat. Place the skillet in a preheated oven.

6. Bake at 400 ° F for about 5-10 minutes or until set.

7. Remove the skillet from the oven and let it rest for a couple of minutes.

8. Cut into 4 equal wedges.

9. Serve 2 wedges in each plate. Top with avocado slices, sriracha sauce, and tomatoes and serve.

Apple Pancakes (Low Carb)

Serves: 4

Nutritional values per serving:

Calories – 117, Fat – 6.2 g, Carbohydrate – 14.5 g, Protein – 1.9 g

Image Courtesy: Pixabay

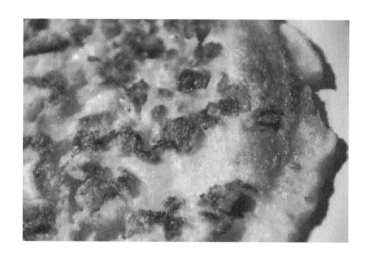

Ingredients:

- ½ tablespoon broken flax

- 6 tablespoons applesauce

- ½ tablespoon maple syrup

- ½ teaspoon ground cinnamon

- ½ teaspoon baking powder

- 3 tablespoons lukewarm water

- ½ cup oatmeal

- 1 tablespoon coconut oil, melted + extra to fry

- ½ tablespoon vanilla extract

- 1/8 teaspoon salt

Method:

1. Add broken flax and lukewarm water into a blender and blend until smooth. Let the mixture sit for 10 minutes in the blender.

2. Add applesauce, maple syrup, ground cinnamon, baking powder, lukewarm water, oatmeal, coconut oil, vanilla extract and salt into the blender. Blend until smooth.

3. If your batter is too thick, add a couple of tablespoons of water and blend again.

4. Pour into a bowl.

5. Place a nonstick pan or griddle over medium heat. Pour about ¼ cup of the batter. Swirl the pan slightly so that the batter spreads.

6. In a while, bubbles will appear on the pancake and the edges will begin to get brown. Flip sides and cook the other

side until golden brown.

7. Follow steps 5-6 and make the remaining pancakes.

8. Serve warm.

Breakfast Egg White Spinach Enchilada Omelets (Low Carb)

Serves: 3

Nutritional values per serving:

Calories – 239, Fat – 12 g, Carbohydrate – 10 g, Protein – 24 g

Image Courtesy: Pixabay

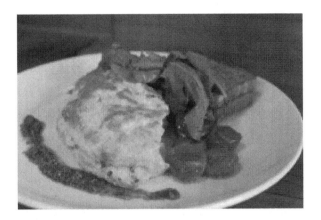

Ingredients:

- 1 ½ cups egg whites or egg whites from 9 large eggs

- Salt to taste

- Pepper to taste

- ¼ cup scallions + extra to garnish

- A handful fresh cilantro, chopped

- ½ can (from a 4.5-ounce can) chopped green chilies

- ¾ cup low fat Colby Jack cheese, grated

- 1 small avocado, peeled, pitted chopped

- 1 tablespoon water

- Cooking spray

- 1 small ripe tomato, diced

- 5 ounces frozen spinach

- Kosher salt to taste

- Freshly ground pepper to taste

- ½ cup green enchilada sauce

Method:

1. Take a small baking dish and spread 3 tablespoons enchilada sauce on the bottom of the dish.

2. Add egg whites, salt, pepper and water into a bowl and whisk well.

3. Place a medium-sized nonstick skillet over medium heat. Spray with cooking spray.

4. When the pan is heated, pour about 1/3 of the egg whites into the pan. Swirl the pan so that the whites spread all over the pan. Cook until the omelet is set.

Flip sides and cook for 40-60 seconds. Carefully slide on to a plate.

5. Repeat the above 2 steps to make the other 2 omelets.

6. Spray some more cooking spray in the pan. Add scallions and sauté until translucent.

7. Stir in tomato, cilantro, and salt and cook for a couple of minutes.

8. Add spinach and green chili. Sauté for a couple of minutes until the spinach wilts.

9. Add pepper to taste. Turn off the heat. Add ¼ cup cheese and stir.

10. Spread the omelets on your countertop. Divide the mixture among the omelets.

11. Roll and place the omelet rolls in the baking dish, with the seam side facing down.

12. Spread remaining enchilada sauce over the rolls. Sprinkle remaining cheese over the rolls.

13. Cover the baking dish with foil.

14. Bake in a preheated oven at 350 ° F for about 15-20 minutes.

15. Sprinkle scallions and avocado on top and serve.

Classic Falafel (Low Carb)

Makes: 12

Nutritional values per serving: 1 falafel without serving options

Calories – 78, Fat – 4 g, Carbohydrate – 8.7 g, Protein – 2.7 g

Image Courtesy: Pixabay

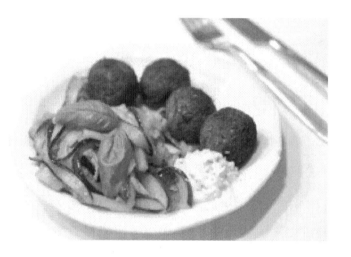

Ingredients:

- ¾ cup dry chickpeas, rinsed
- ¼ cup white onion, finely chopped
- 1 tablespoon oat flour
- ½ tablespoon cumin powder
- ½ teaspoon coriander powder
- A pinch cardamom powder
- Cayenne pepper to taste (optional)
- ¼ cup fresh parsley, chopped
- 3 cloves garlic, minced

- Salt to taste

- Grape seed oil or any other oil to fry

Method:

1. Place chickpeas into a pot. Pour enough water to cover the chickpeas by about 2 inches.

2. Place the pot over high heat. When the water begins to boil, let it boil for a couple of minutes. Turn off the heat. Cover and set aside for an hour.

3. Drain and rinse again. Cook the beans in a pressure cooker or instant pot by covering with water. You can also cook in a pot. Cook until soft.

4. Drain and cool the chickpeas. Transfer into a food processor bowl. Process until finely chopped.

5. Add onion, parsley and garlic and pulse until well combined. Add oat flour, cumin, coriander, salt and cayenne pepper and pulse until well combined. Scrape the sides of the food processor if

required.

6. Taste and adjust the salt and spices if necessary. Transfer into a bowl. Cover and chill for an hour. If the mixture is very moist, add some more oat flour. If too dry, process for some more time in the food processor with a sprinkle of water.

7. Divide the mixture into 12 equal portions. Shape into patties.

8. Place a nonstick pan or griddle over medium heat. Add a little oil. Swirl the pan to spread the oil. Fry the falafel in batches.

9. Cook until the underside is golden brown. Flip sides and cook the other side until golden brown.

10. Remove with a slotted spoon and place on a plate lined with paper towels.

11. Serve with pita bread or greens. You can also serve with a low carb dip of your choice.

Parsley and Garlic Chicken Cutlets with Broccoli (Low Carb)

Serves: 4

Nutritional values per serving: 12.4 ounces

Calories – 486, Fat – 19 g, Carbohydrate – 15.7 g, Protein – 54 g

Image Courtesy: Pixabay

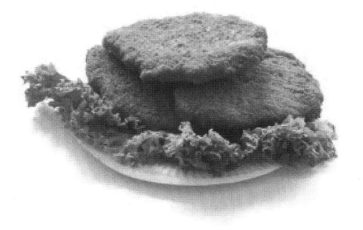

Ingredients:

- 8 organic chicken cutlets (about 6-8 ounces each)

- 2 ½ tablespoons olive oil

- 5-6 tablespoons whole wheat pastry flour

- 10 tablespoons dry white wine

- 3 cloves garlic, chopped

- Sea salt to taste

- 1 ½ tablespoons butter, cut into small pieces

- 3 tablespoons fresh parsley, chopped

- 15 ounces fresh broccoli florets

Method:

1. Place flour in a shallow bowl. Dredge the chicken cutlets in the flour.

2. Place a nonstick skillet over medium-high heat. Add half the oil. When the oil

is heated, place a few of the cutlets (cook the remaining in batches). Cook for 3-5 minutes. Flip sides and cook for 3-5 minutes.

3. Meanwhile, add cauliflower into a microwave safe bowl. Microwave on High until tender. It should take 6-7 minutes.

4. Remove the chicken with a slotted spoon and place on a plate lined with paper towels.

5. Add garlic into the same skillet. Sauté until aromatic. Stir in the wine and let it simmer until it is half its original quantity.

6. Remove from heat and stir in the butter, salt, and parsley.

7. Place 2 cutlets in each plate. Pour the butter sauce over it. Place broccoli alongside and serve.

Avocado Ranch Chicken Salad (Low Carb)

Serves: 3

Nutritional values per serving: 2/3 cup

Calories – 361, Fat – 23 g, Carbohydrate – 5 g, Protein – 32 g

Image Courtesy: Pixabay

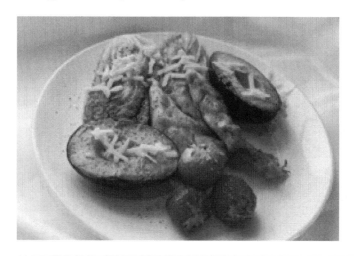

Ingredients:

- 1 medium ripe avocado, peeled, pitted, scooped

- 1 tablespoon chopped pickled jalapeño

- Salt to taste

- 1 ½ cups shredded or chopped cooked chicken

- 2 tablespoons finely chopped onions

- ¼ cup low carb ranch dressing

- ½ tablespoons white wine vinegar

- Pepper to taste

- ¼ cup celery, chopped

Method:

1. Add avocado, jalapeño, salt, ranch dressing, vinegar and pepper into the food processor. Process until smooth. Pour into a bowl.

2. Add chicken, red onion and celery into the bowl and fold gently.

3. Serve as is or chill for a couple of hours and serve later.

Grilled Salmon and Vegetables (Low Carb)

Serves: 2

Nutritional values per serving: 1 salmon piece with 1 ¼ cups vegetable

Calories – 281, Fat – 13 g, Carbohydrate – 11 g, Protein – 30 g

Image Courtesy: Pixabay

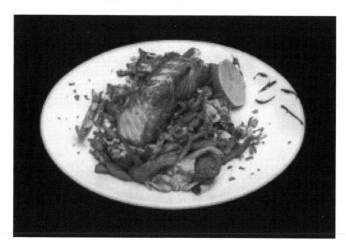

Ingredients:

- 1 small zucchini, halved lengthwise

- 1 small red onion, cut into 1-inch wedges

- Salt to taste

- 10 ounces salmon fillets, cut into 2 equal portions

- Lemon wedges to serve

- 1 bell pepper of any color, trimmed, halved, deseeded

- ½ tablespoon extra-virgin olive oil

- Pepper to taste

- A handful fresh basil, sliced

Method:

1. Brush a little oil over onion, bell pepper, and zucchini. Season with salt.

2. Season salmon with salt and pepper.

3. Place all the vegetables and salmon on a preheated grill (place the salmon skin side facing down). Cook the vegetables for 4-6 minutes on each side or until done. Do not turn the salmon while it is cooking. Remove the vegetables and salmon from the grill as it cooks.

4. Place the vegetables on your cutting

board. When cool enough to handle, chop into smaller pieces.

5. Place the vegetables in a bowl. Toss well. Discard the skin from the salmon.

6. Serve salmon with vegetables garnished with basil and lemon wedges.

Steak Tacos (High Carb)

Serves: 2

Nutritional values per serving: 2 tacos, without toppings

Calories – 325, Fat – 7 g, Carbohydrate – 29 g, Protein – 37 g

Image Courtesy: Pixabay

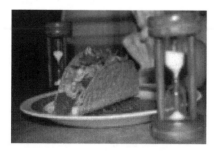

Ingredients:

- Juice of a lime
- ½ teaspoon chili powder
- ¼ teaspoon paprika
- ¼ teaspoon onion powder
- ¼ teaspoon dried oregano
- 4 corn tortillas
- 2 tablespoons chopped onions
- ½ teaspoon salt
- ¼ teaspoon cumin powder
- ¼ teaspoon garlic powder
- Pepper to taste
- 2/3 pound lean sirloin steak, trimmed of fat
- A handful fresh cilantro, chopped
- ¼ cup salsa
- ½ tablespoon oil

Method:

1. Add chili powder, lime juice, paprika, onion powder, oregano, salt, cumin powder, garlic powder and pepper into a bowl. Mix well.

2. Rub this mixture over the steak.

3. Grill the steak on a preheated grill for 5-6 minutes on each side for medium-rare or the way you like it cooked.

4. When done, place on your cutting board. When cool enough to handle, cut into smaller pieces.

5. Place a skillet over medium heat. Place a skillet over medium heat. Add oil. When the oil is heated, add the chopped steak and sauté for 4-5 minutes.

6. Warm the tortillas following the instructions on the package.

7. Spread the tortillas on your countertop. Place the steak on the tortillas. Garnish with cilantro and any other toppings of your choice if desired. Roll and serve.

Asian Beef Zoodle Soup (Low Carb)

Serves: 2

Nutritional values per serving:

Calories −241, Fat − 8.5 g, Carbohydrate − 19.5 g, Protein − 23 g

Image Courtesy: Pixabay

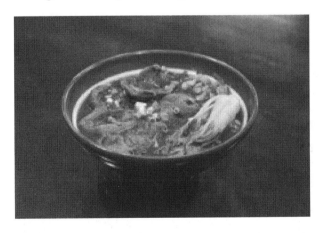

Ingredients:

- ½ tablespoon coconut oil

- 3 ounces fresh shiitake mushrooms,

sliced

- 1 teaspoon fresh ginger, minced

- 1 tablespoon coconut aminos

- ½ teaspoon kosher salt

- 6 ounces beef sirloin steak, boneless, cut into thin slices, across the grain

- ½ small onion, halved, thinly sliced

- 1 clove garlic, minced

- 2 ½ cups beef bone broth

- 1 teaspoon Red Boat fish sauce

- 1 medium zucchini

For toppings:

- A handful fresh cilantro, chopped

- A handful fresh basil, chopped

- Lime wedges

- 2 tablespoons thinly sliced green onion

- ½ jalapeño, thinly sliced

Method:

1. Place a soup pot over medium heat. Add oil. When the oil melts, add onion and sauté until translucent.

2. Stir in the mushrooms and cook for a couple of minutes. Stir in the ginger and garlic and sauté for a few seconds until aromatic.

3. Stir in the broth, fish sauce, coconut aminos, and salt.

4. When it begins to boil, lower the heat to medium low and let it simmer for 4-5 minutes.

5. Meanwhile, make noodles of the zucchini (zoodles) using a spiralizer or a julienne peeler.

6. Add zoodles into the pot and cook for a couple of minutes until slightly tender.

7. Add steak and stir. Let it simmer for a minute.

8. Serve topped with cilantro, basil, green onion, jalapeño and lemon wedges.

Chicken and Zucchini Burgers (Low Carb)

Serves: 8

Nutritional values per serving: Without toppings and bun

Calories – 268, Fat – 13 g, Carbohydrate – 5 g, Protein – 34 g

Image Courtesy: Pixabay

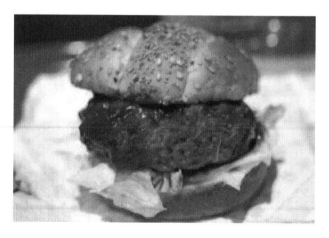

Ingredients:

- 2 zucchinis, grated

- 1 cup ricotta cheese

- 2 teaspoons garlic powder

- 2 teaspoons kosher salt or to taste

- 1 teaspoon pepper

- 2 pounds 99% lean ground chicken

- 2 eggs

- 2 teaspoons Italian seasoning

- 1 teaspoon onion powder

- 2 tablespoons olive oil

Method:

1. Place zucchini in a colander. Sprinkle salt and mix. Let it remain in the colander for 10-15 minutes.

2. Squeeze the zucchini of excess moisture using cheesecloth.

3. Place in a bowl. Add ricotta, garlic powder, pepper, chicken, eggs, seasoning and onion powder into the bowl. Mix well. Divide the mixture into

8 equal portions. Shape into burgers.

4. Place a skillet over medium heat. Add half the oil. Place 4 burgers. Cook until the underside is golden brown. Flip sides and cook the other side until golden brown and burger cooked through.

5. Repeat the previous step and cook the remaining burgers.

6. Alternately, you can grill the burgers on a preheated grill.

7. Serve with toppings of your choice or in a low carb bun.

Swedish Meatballs (Low Carb)

Serves: 8

Nutritional values per serving: 5 meatballs without noodles

Calories – 213.5, Fat – 10 g, Carbohydrate – 8.5 g, Protein – 25.1 g

Image Courtesy: Pixabay

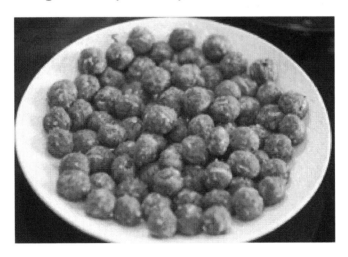

Ingredients:

- 2 teaspoons olive oil
- 2 cloves garlic, minced
- ½ cup parsley, minced
- 2 large eggs
- Salt to taste
- Pepper to taste
- 4 cups beef stock
- 2 small onions, minced
- 2 stalks celery, minced
- 2 pounds 93% lean ground beef
- ½ cup seasoned breadcrumbs
- 1 teaspoon ground allspice
- 4 ounces light cream cheese

Method:

1. Place a skillet over medium heat. Add

oil. When the oil is heated, add garlic and onion and sauté until soft.

2. Stir in the parsley and celery and sauté until soft. Turn off the heat and cool for a while. Transfer into a large bowl.

3. Add beef, breadcrumbs, pepper, salt, allspice, and eggs into the bowl of onions. Mix well.

4. Divide the mixture into 40 equal portions and shape into balls.

5. Pour beef stock into the skillet. Place the skillet over medium heat. When it begins to boil, carefully add meatballs into the broth. Cover the skillet with a lid.

6. Carefully remove the meatballs using a slotted spoon and place in a bowl.

7. Pass the stock through a strainer placed over a bowl. Pour the stock into a blender. Add cream cheese and blend until smooth.

8. Pour it back into the skillet. Place the skillet over medium heat. Let the sauce thicken slightly.

9. Pour the sauce into the bowl of meatballs. Stir lightly.

10. Sprinkle parsley and serve as it is or with low carb noodles.

Shrimp Scampi over Zoodles (Low Carb)

Serves: 4

Nutritional values per serving: 6 shrimp and ¼ the zoodles

Calories – 170, Fat – 7 g, Carbohydrate – 12 g, Protein – 11 g

Image Courtesy: Pixabay

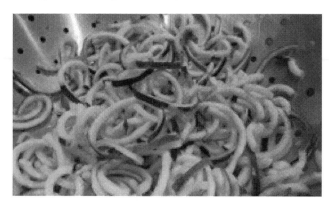

Ingredients:

- 4 large zucchinis, trimmed

- 4 teaspoons garlic, minced

- 24 large shrimp, shelled, deveined

- 3 tablespoons fresh lemon juice

- 4 tablespoons low-fat butter or Smart balance light

- ¼ teaspoon crushed red pepper flakes (optional)

- 5 tablespoons white wine or low sodium chicken broth

- 4 teaspoons parmesan cheese, grated

- Salt to taste

- Pepper to taste

Method:

1. Make noodles of the zucchini (zoodles) using a spiralizer or a julienne peeler.

2. Add zoodles into a microwavable bowl.

Microwave on High for 2 minutes or until tender.

3. Place a large nonstick pan over medium-low heat. Add butter. When butter melts, add garlic and red pepper flakes and sauté until aromatic. Stir constantly.

4. Stir in the shrimp and sauté until pink. Sprinkle salt and pepper. Remove shrimp with a slotted spoon and place in a bowl.

5. Raise the heat to medium heat. Pour white wine and lemon juice into the pan. Scrape the bottom of the pan to remove any browned bits that may have stuck. Simmer for 2-3 minutes.

6. Stir in the zoodles and shrimp. Mix well. Heat thoroughly.

7. Divide equally the zoodles among 4 plates. Place 6 shrimp on each plate.

8. Sprinkle 1-teaspoon cheese on each plate and serve.

Almond Crusted Pork Tenders

(Low Carb)

Serves: 8

Nutritional values per serving:

Calories – 293, Fat – 13 g, Carbohydrate – 5 g, Protein – 38 g

Image Courtesy: Pixabay

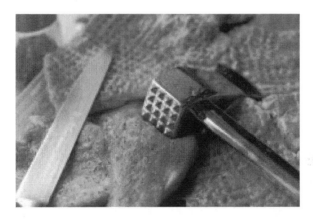

Ingredients:

- 2 2/3 pounds lean pork tenderloin, cut into ½ inch thick round slices
- 1 cup almond meal

- 4 teaspoons paprika

- 1 teaspoon salt

- Cooking spray

- 4 egg whites

- ½ cup almonds, sliced

- 1 teaspoon garlic powder

- 1 teaspoon pepper

Method:

1. Add whites into a wide bowl. Whisk well. Place almond meal, paprika, almonds, salt, garlic powder and pepper in another wide bowl and stir.

2. First, dip the pork slices in whites. Shake to drop off excess egg. Next dredge in almond meal mixture. Place on a wire rack. Place the wire rack on a baking sheet. Spray cooking spray over the pork on both the sides.

3. Place the baking sheet in the oven.

4. Bake in a preheated oven at 425 ° F for

about 15-20 minutes or until cooked through. Broil for the last couple of minutes if you want a crunchy top.

5. Serve.

Turkey Moussaka (Low Carb)

Serves: 8

Nutritional values per serving:

Calories – 385, Fat – 16 g, Carbohydrate – 22 g, Protein – 38 g

Image Courtesy: Pixabay

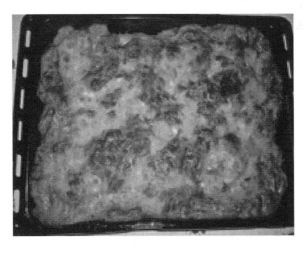

Ingredients:

- 4 eggplants, cut into ½ inch rounds

- 2 pounds 93% lean ground turkey

- 8 cloves garlic, minced

- 1 cup red wine

- ½ teaspoon ground nutmeg

- ¼ cup parsley, chopped

- 2/3 cup parmesan cheese, grated

- 4 teaspoons extra-virgin olive oil

- 1 large yellow onion, chopped

- 4 tablespoons tomato paste

- ½ teaspoon ground cinnamon

- 24 ounces fat-free Greek yogurt

- 2 eggs

- Salt to taste

- Pepper to taste

Method:

1. Line a large baking sheet with parchment paper. Spray with cooking spray. Lay the eggplant slices in one layer without overlapping. Roast in batches if required.

2. Spray cooking spray on top of the eggplant slices. Sprinkle salt and pepper.

3. Bake in a preheated oven at 425 ° F for about 5-10 minutes or until light brown. Remove from the oven.

4. Add yogurt, cheese, eggs, half the parsley, salt and pepper into a bowl. Mix well.

5. Place a nonstick skillet over medium-high heat. Add oil. When the oil is heated, add onion and garlic and sauté until soft.

6. Add turkey, salt, and pepper. Sauté until brown.

7. Stir in the nutmeg, cinnamon and tomato paste. Mix until well combined.

8. Pour red wine and stir. Let it cook for

4-5 minutes.

9. Grease a casserole dish with cooking spray. Place eggplant slices on the bottom of the dish. Layer with turkey mixture. Spread it evenly. Spread yogurt mixture evenly on top.

10. Bake in a preheated oven at 425 ° F for about 20 – 30 minutes or until the top is browned as per your liking.

11. Remove from the oven. Cool for a while and serve.

Creamy Cajun Chicken Pasta (Low Carb)

Serves: 8

Nutritional values per serving: 2 cups

Calories – 344, Fat – 10 g, Carbohydrate – 23 g, Protein – 37 g

Image Courtesy: Pixabay

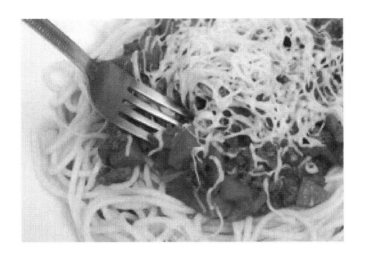

Ingredients:

- 2 spaghetti squashes, halved, deseeded

- 4 tablespoons Cajun seasoning, divided or more to taste

- 2 green bell peppers, thinly sliced

- 2 red bell peppers, thinly sliced

- 1 red onion, thinly sliced

- 2 cans (14 ounces each) fire-roasted diced tomatoes with its liquid

- ½ cup scallions

- 2 2/3 pounds chicken breast, skinless, boneless, chopped into chunks

- 4 teaspoons olive oil

- 4-6 cloves garlic, minced

- 1 cup low fat cream cheese

Method:

1. Spray the cut part of the spaghetti squash halves with cooking spray. Cover each of the squash halves with foil. Place the squash halves on a baking sheet.

2. Bake in a preheated oven at 375 ° F for about 45-60 minutes or until tender.

3. When done, unwrap and cool for a while. When cool enough to handle, scrape the flesh of the squash with a fork. Place in a bowl. Discard the outer covering of the squash.

4. Place chicken in a bowl. Sprinkle half the Cajun seasoning over the chicken and toss well. Place a large skillet over medium heat. Add oil. When the oil is heated, add chicken. Sauté until tender.

5. Add bell peppers and onion and sauté for 3-4 minutes.

6. Lower the heat to low heat. Stir in the tomatoes, half the Cajun seasoning, and cream cheese.

7. When the cream cheese melts, turn off the heat. Taste and adjust salt and pepper if required.

8. Add chicken and shredded spaghetti squash. Toss well.

9. Garnish with scallions and serve.

Thai Green Curry (Low Carb)

Serves: 4

Nutritional values per serving: Without rice

Calories – 380, Fat – 32.4 g, Carbohydrate – 18.5 g, Protein – 9.4 g

Image Courtesy: Pixabay

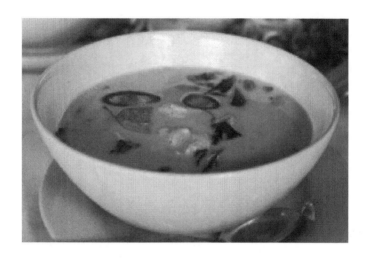

Ingredients:

For green curry:

- 1 sweet potato, peeled, cut into cubes

- 1 ½ cups broccoli florets

- 1 ½ cans (14 ounces each) coconut milk

- 2 teaspoons olive oil

- Salt to taste

- 2 tablespoons Thai green curry paste

- 24 ounces firm tofu

Optional:

- 1 tablespoon golden raisins

- A handful fresh cilantro, chopped

- A dash of fish sauce

- Brown sugar to taste

- Cooked rice

Method:

1. Press the tofu of excess moisture using paper towels. Chop into cubes.

2. Place a soup pot over medium-high heat. Add oil. When the oil is heated, add tofu and salt and sauté until brown. Remove tofu with a slotted spoon and set aside.

3. Place the pot back over heat. Add coconut milk and curry paste and stir until well combined. Add sweet potatoes and cook until tender.

4. Stir in the broccoli and tofu cook for 3-4 minutes or until broccoli is crisp as well as tender.

5. Add the optional ingredients if using and stir.

6. Serve with rice.

Tofu Vegetables Noodle Bowl

Serves: 6

Nutritional values per serving:

Calories – 344, Fat – 21 g, Carbohydrate – 26 g, Protein – 17 g

Image Courtesy: Pixabay

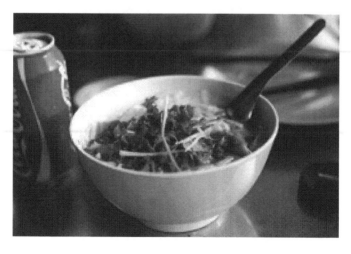

Ingredients:

- 24 ounces extra firm tofu

- 2 tablespoons low sodium tamari

- 2 tablespoons rice wine vinegar

- 3 tablespoons coconut oil

- 2 tablespoons garlic, peeled, minced

- 1 pound cabbage, thinly sliced (about 10 cups after slicing)

- 4 carrots, peeled, cut into thin strips

- 1 green bell pepper, deseeded, cut into thin strips

- 1 yellow or red bell pepper, deseeded, cut into thin strips

- ½ cup walnuts, roughly chopped

- Freshly ground pepper to taste

- 1 cup vegetable stock

- 1 teaspoon maple syrup

- 2 teaspoons sesame oil

- 2 tablespoons ginger, peeled, minced

- 1 large head broccoli, cut into bite-size florets (about 4 cups florets)

- Sea salt to taste

Method:

1. Press the tofu of excess moisture using paper towels. You can also place a heavy bottomed pan over the tofu to drain the excess moisture.

2. Add stock, maple syrup, tamari, rice wine vinegar and sesame oil into a bowl and mix until well combined.

3. Place a large wok or skillet over high heat. Add 2 tablespoons oil. When the oil is heated, add tofu and cook until golden brown on all the sides. Remove with a slotted spoon and set aside on a plate lined with paper towels.

4. Add 1-tablespoon oil. When the oil is heated, add ginger and garlic and sauté for a few seconds until aromatic. Stir in the bell peppers, broccoli, and carrots.

Cook for a couple of minutes.

5. Add cabbage and sauté for a minute. Season with salt and pepper. Cook for a couple of minutes.

6. Add tofu back into the skillet. Mix well. Add walnuts and the stock mixture. Mix well. Cook until nearly dry.

7. Turn off the heat.

8. Spoon into bowls and serve hot.

Conclusion

I want to thank you once again for purchasing this book. I hope it proved to be an informative and interesting read.

Carb cycling is a simple diet plan and it is quite versatile. You can tweak it to meet your needs. The only rule of carb cycling that you need to follow is to alternate between days of the high, moderate, and low carb intake. As long as you stick to this pattern, you will see a positive change in your body and health. You will not only be able to lose weight and fat, but you will also be able to maintain the weight loss with this incredible diet.

Follow the simple rules provided in this book to create a carb cycling diet that meets all your requirements. The sample meal plan along with the recipes given in this book will enable you to kickstart the process of carb cycling to achieve your weight loss and fitness goals. All the recipes curated in this book are quite easy to follow and simple to cook. You will be able to cook tasty and nutritious food within no time. The one thing that you must be mindful of is the number of carbs that you consume. Follow the simple tips given and you are good to go. Now, all that you need to do is follow the protocols of carb cycling and achieve your fitness goals.

Thank you and all the best!

Sources

https://www.myprotein.com/thezone/nutrition/the-benefits-of-carb-cycling/

https://draxe.com/carb-cycling-diet/

https://www.bodybuilding.com/content/carbohydrate-cycling-what-you-need-to-know.html

https://www.oxygenmag.com/nutrition/erin-sterns-top-5-tips-for-carb-cycling#gid=ci02285cd4a000244c&pid=shutterstock_794250856

Made in the USA
Columbia, SC
10 January 2019